CATARRH, COLDS AND GRIPPE

CATARRH, COLDS AND GRIPPE

Including Prevention and Cure,

With Chapters on
Nasal Polypus,
Hay Fever and
Influenza,

BY

JOHN H. CLARKE, M.D.,

GYAN

Published by

Gyan Publishing House
5, Ansari Road
Daryaganj, New Delhi-110002
Phone: 011-47034999, 9811692060
E-mail: books@gyanbooks.com

Distribution Network
gyanbooks.com
India, USA, Canada, UK, Australia, France

ISBN : 978-81-212-6597-3 (PB)
First Published, 1899

2nd Impression 2022

Printed at: Gyan Press, Delhi.

CATARRH, COLDS AND GRIPPE
Author: JOHN H. CLARKE

Catarrh, Colds and Grippe,

Including Prevention and Cure,

**With Chapters on
Nasal Polypus,
Hay Fever and
Influenza,**

BY

JOHN H. CLARKE, M. D.,

Consulting Physician to the London Homœopathic Hospital; Editor of the "Homœopathic World;" Author of "The Prescriber," "A Dictionary of Domestic Medicine," "Indigestion: Its Causes and Cure;" "A Bird's-eye View of the Homœopathic System of Medicine," Etc.

AMERICAN EDITION.

Revised by the Author from the Fourth English Edition.

1899.

CONTENTS.

PREFACE TO AMERICAN EDITION.

An extensive experience among American residents and visitors in London convinces me that among the bonds of community between the two great divisions of Anglo-Saxonia, one of no little importance is a common interest in the sub ject of nasal catarrh. I must, therefore, abandon the claim I made in the first editions of this work, that "cold in the head" is a British interest *par excellence;* and in offering this little work to American readers I trust that my insular standpoint will prove no bar to its wider usefulness.

JOHN H. CLARKE.

30 Clarges Street,

Piccadilly, London W.,

July, 1899.

PREFACE TO FOURTH ENGLISH EDITION.

THE call for a new edition of my little treatise on COLDS has enabled me to put it through a complete revision, and at the same time to add a section on that most unwelcome visitor of recent years—EPIDEMIC INFLUENZA. The name *Influenza* has become indissolubly connected with colds in the head; and epidemic influenza has so many features in common with ordinary colds, that some account of the malady and how it may be cured, together with the large family of ills it leaves behind it, seems called for in the present volume.

I have heard many people say in reference to the scourge, which is now in the seventh year of its visitation, that it is ridiculous to call *this* INFLUENZA: *this* is something a great deal worse! But, as a matter of fact, the epidemic influenza is the originator of the name, severe colds having been called "influenza colds" after it.

For centuries the epidemic disease has prevailed in Western Europe at uncertain intervals, and for want of a more definite description the Italians named it "Influenza," or "The Influence." And as this name does not commit any one to special views as to the pathology of the disease, it is so far unobjectionable, and has become generally adopted.

My own theory as to the application of the name to severe ordinary colds is this: For some time after a visitation of an epidemic, infectious colds of a severe type have prevailed, and have been called "Influenza Colds," to distinguish them from common non-infectious colds. By degrees, for the sake of shortness, they have been called simply "Influenza." Hence has arisen the confusion when the next epidemic has come round.

The name our French neighbours have given it is "La Grippe," which is sufficiently suggestive of the sudden manner in which it seizes its victims, and this term, in its Anglified form of "grip," is the favourite name of the disease on the American Continent.

I have also taken the opportunity of adding a chapter on a frequent consequence and concomitant of chronic colds, NASAL POLYPUS; and another on HAY FEVER; and I have given an account of some remedies not mentioned in the earlier editions, including an important remedy, newly introduced by Dr. Cooper, *Lemna minor*.

JOHN H. CLARKE.

FROM THE

PREFACES TO THE FIRST AND SECOND EDITIONS.

My subject is discussed under three main heads,—Cold-Catching, Cold-Preventing, and Cold-Curing. The prevention and cure of colds are partly medicinal and partly general. It is possible to cure colds or prevent them by general measures, and these will be referred to in detail. But medicines are the most powerful agents we possess both in dealing with colds when taken, and in fortifying the constitution against their recurrence. The last portion of my work will be devoted to this section;

and I shall add a short *Materia Medica*, in which the Medicines most suitable for colds will be arranged in alphabetical order, and their particular properties and indications for use described.

When I first sent this little work to the public, I urged on its behalf that the COMMON COLD IN THE HEAD had never before possessed a treatise devoted entirely to itself; and I maintained that it deserved one just as much as other more dignified diseases. My plea has been accepted in the most satisfactory way; for within three months of the book's first appearance, I have been asked by the publishers to prepare a second edition. The COMMON COLD has thus triumphantly vindicated its right to be deemed a serious disease in the estimation of the British public.

I am not sure that even a higher distinction might not be claimed for it, namely, to be called "*The* British disease" *par excellence*. Foreigners, as is well known, reserve that name for what they call "the spleen," meaning by this, low spirits, melancholy, and tendency to suicide, which they attribute to our foggy climate. Naturally we British are not so keenly alive to the prevalence and gravity of "the spleen" as our observant neighbours; but there is no denying that we do possess peculiar facilities for catching cold. I venture to think (as I shall explain in my introductory chapter) that the prevalence of colds has something to do with the melancholy temper which foreigners think so distinctive of the British nation, and is the real explanation of that mysterious affection "the spleen." The "spleen," I may remark, is not recognized by medical men as a disease at all, but only as an inoffensive organ of the body. But our colds are acknowledged by everybody—doctors, laity, and foreigners—and if we have a distinctively national disease at all, I should certainly give this name to COLD IN THE HEAD.

JOHN H. CLARKE.

Catarrh, Colds and Grippe.

CHAPTER I.

COLDS.

VERY little sympathy is bestowed on an unfortunate who has taken a cold in his head. It is a humiliating thing, and he feels it. Also, what is worse, his friends share his feeling, and despise him (secretly, of course) as much as he despises himself, and vote him a nuisance. It must have been mere stupidity on his part, they feel, that made him catch the cold—if it was not sheer malice—just on purpose to annoy them with his sneezings and continual nose-moppings. Now, if the chill he had taken had only gone to his lungs, and laid him up with pneumonia, the same friends would have been all sympathy and devotion, and the doctor would have been summoned post-haste. And yet the misery, though not the danger, of a cold in the head is quite as great as that of pneumonia, and generally lasts much longer, and the victim is no less deserving of sympathy in the former case than in the latter.

Besides the humiliation, a cold is such a waster of time. Whatever a man may be doing, every few minutes his nose must be attended to and his eyes wiped before the work can be gone on with. An artist at his easel, or an author at his desk, must drop pen or brush every little while, whatever may be the high inspirations that are crying within for utterance. Finally, there is the depression that some sufferers feel when seized with a cold in the head. It is sometimes quite terrible. Life is not worth living for them; and I should not be surprised if the true explanation of the many inscrutable cases of suicide we read of in the papers was not to be found in this as, at least, a partial cause. When the combined wisdom of jury and coroner can assign "no cause for the rash act," it might help them to something definite if they were to ask whether the deceased had not had a severe cold in his head at the time.

We speak of a cold in the head as if there was only one kind of cold; but the fact is, there is an infinite variety. Every person almost has something characteristic about the course and progress of his unassisted cold. The orthodox cold is the one which begins, after sitting in a draught, with a creeping chilly feeling up the back, culminating in a sneeze. Then there is a lull in the proceedings; but the nose never feels quite easy, and by-and-by another sneeze announces that the damage is really done. Soon a "Contest between the Eyes and

Nose" sets in as to which can run the fastest; then the running slackens, the nose becomes stopped by swelling of mucous membrane, which afterwards relieves itself by giving off a thick secretion. But for days there is a general susceptibility. The faintest airs are felt as thorough draughts and set the patient off sneezing. He can't get away from the thought of his nose, try how he will. It is the last thing he thinks of at night, and the first thing that claims his thoughts in the morning; and this goes on indefinitely, depending much on the time of the year, the state of the weather, and the treatment he receives. Sometimes, in spite of everything, it goes on day after day until he begins to think it will really never end.

This is the orthodox cold. But all colds are not orthodox. Very often the first thing to announce a cold is the sneeze, no preliminary chill having been felt. And, again, some people begin to feel a cold first in the throat, and it gradually works its way upwards and forwards.

The influenza cold I do not rank as a distinct variety. It is the fashion to call very severe colds "influenza," and to attribute them to the prevalence of "ozone clouds." Certain it is that colds do prevail in epidemic fashion, and at times seem to come independently of any distinct chill. But once taken, the cold is indistinguishable from any other severe cold by its characteristics.

There is also the "catching" cold; for some colds, at any rate, are infectious. It is well known that when a cold of this description once appears in a family—often first in the person of the domestic cat—it "goes through the house," every member of that household feeling its effects sooner or later.

Epidemic influenza (which is also infectious) I shall deal with later on, in a section by itself. The name of the disease, and the way in which it became associated with ordinary colds, I have already discussed in the preface to this volume.

This is an inquiring age, and doubtless the question will be put to me—What *is* a cold in the head? The principal feature is a swollen and congested condition of the mucous membrane lining the nostrils and the air spaces connected with them, with increased irritability of the membrane and increased and altered secretion. The "full" sensation in the head is due to extension of the swelling along the offshoots of the nasal mucous membrane, which line the cavities in the skull bones,—those, for instance, which lie in the frontal bone, where it forms the prominences of the eyebrows. The deafness which sometimes accompanies a cold in the head depends on swelling of the mucous membrane which lines the tube passing from the back of the nose to the ear. The chilliness and sensitiveness of the skin which accompany cold in the head indicate that the affection is constitutional as well as local, and show that some change has been brought about in the vital resisting power.

Snuff or pepper will make a person sneeze, and set up mucous secretion for the time; but in this case the action is local only and not constitutional, and no cold has really been taken, though the symptoms, as far as the nose is concerned, are identical. It is this fact of the constitutional character of a cold that makes the selection of the remedy often a matter of some difficulty. The cold medicines, such as *Aconite*, *Arsenicum*, and *Mercurius*, each affect the system generally as well as locally, and cause all the constitutional symptoms of cold, and yet all differently from one another. Consequently, in choosing a remedy for cold, we must bear in mind the constitutional symptoms of the patient and the constitutional symptoms of the drugs.

The simple irritation of the nasal mucous membrane, with slight mucous secretion often experienced in the beginning of cold weather, does not constitute cold. It is analogous to the chapping of the hands, and is purely a local effect.

In some instances one attack of

cold appears to be protective against other attacks. A person has regularly at the beginning of winter one cold. This, in a week or two, is got over, and then he goes the rest of the year round without having another attack.

Having said this much regarding the pathology of Cold in the Head, we can say little more. Why chilling of the surface of the body should sometimes be followed by all this train of symptoms is one of the many points in medical affairs still in the region of speculation. The *Lancet* the other day promised us that, "thanks to the researches of German experimenters," "scientific doctors" might hope to be able, "in the near future," to tell whether any given stomach was out of order or not. At present we know pretty well whether we have a cold in the head or not without the assistance of a "scientific physician;" but if these German experimenters take up the subject of a Cold in the Head, it is possible that "in the near future" we shall be unable to have scientific assurance even of that. Let us hope they will leave it alone. For our purposes it is enough to know when we have got a cold, how to cure it when we have got it, and how to avoid getting another.

CHAPTER II.

COLD-CATCHING.

THERE are innumerable ways of catching cold, and some people are peculiarly expert in the art. They will pick up a cold when ordinary people would not have experienced the slightest change of temperature or movement of air. Perhaps the commonest way of taking cold is by sitting in a draught, especially if the sitter is either heated in any way, tired, or exhausted. But it does not need chilling of the whole body; and some people are vulnerable in one part and some in another. Most people are liable to cold if they get their feet wet and chilled; but some are more sensitive in the hands, and if driving or walking without gloves on a rainy day, will have a cold in the head developed forthwith. It is by no means necessary to have a draught in order to catch cold. It is quite sufficient to sit near a closed window, on a cold day, glass forming an insufficient protection against the cold without; or even to sit in a cold room away from a window. This is one of the penalties that occasionally attend making morning calls. The caller is shown into a room kept for the purpose, the sunshine being excluded for fear of damage to the carpets, and the windows kept perpetually closed for fear of dust. A room of this kind is like a well, even in the height of summer, and many a cold has been caught in warm weather by a twenty-minutes' stay in such an atmosphere. But it is not cold rooms alone that give cold. There are persons who take cold from going into a room that is over-heated, and begin to sneeze and show signs of catarrh almost as soon as they enter. On the other hand, there is the very common way of taking cold by going out of a heated room into the cold air with insufficient wraps.

Some people seem to have a mania for changing their clothes.

They will leave off a warm garment on a cold day out of pure caprice. Others will put on their summer clothing on a sunny morning in March, and be caught in a snowstorm before the day is over. The only persons who are astonished when these catch cold are their innocent selves.

Sleeping in damp sheets is a frequent cause of taking cold, but generally it is something worse than a cold in the head that follows this. It is a most dangerous thing to do, and when the choice lies between a damp bed or none, the latter should be unhesitatingly chosen. During sleep, the resisting power of the body is at its lowest ebb, and damp clothing at any time will drain off the vital force, and therefore much more certainly when the person is asleep. Very dangerous, also, though not quite so dangerous as sleeping in damp sheets, is wearing insufficiently aired underlinen. Many violent chills are taken in this way, and also through sitting in wet clothes, after being out in the rain, especially if heated at the time; dry clothes should always be put on before sitting down to rest.

Excessive indulgence in cold water is sometimes answerable for colds. "The Englishman's stupid devotion to his morning tub," I once heard a French doctor say, "is the cause of a great deal of his rheumatism and other diseases which are the effects of cold." And though some of my readers may be inclined to vote him right off "a nasty, dirty thing," there was some truth in his criticism. And, indeed, he is an impartial witness, as he is himself a bath-doctor, being resident physician at one of the great continental bathing establishments. There are some people, mostly young men, who think it quite necessary to wash their heads in cold water every morning, and quite unnecessary to dry them. This, they think, clears their brains, and saves them the necessity of using bear's grease—the hair when wet lying flat and straight without it. The human organism is really very accommodating, and will sometimes bear even this treatment without resenting it. But not always; for many a violent cold is taken in this way.

The morning cold bath is an excellent institution when it is judiciously used. For persons in vigorous health, with good circulations and freely acting skins, nothing is more wholesome than the morning tub and scrub-down with a rough towel afterwards. This is one of the best means of fortifying the system against the effects of chill. But like many other good things in this world, the bath-room is not an unmixed boon. Apart from the possibility of the cistern getting out of order, and the servant dropping a paraffin lamp into it in an endeavour to find out what is wrong, there are other risks attending this latest necessity of the modern house.

The human skin is a complex organ. It covers in all the other organs; but besides acting as a covering, it contains many structures within itself. There are the sweat glands, the hair follicles, and the sebaceous glands, secreting an oily matter which keeps the skin soft, and prevents the too rapid removal of the outer particles of the scarf-skin. The scarf-skin is composed of a number of layers of microscopic cells, round in the deeper parts, flat, like scales, on the surface. The surface scales are constantly coming away, and making room for the new cells beneath.

When the skin is in a healthy condition, this scaling-off is imperceptible, except, perhaps, on the head.

Some skins are poor in the secretion of the sebaceous glands. The consequence of this is that these skins are more susceptible to outside influences, as the secretion, besides giving softness to the skin, gives it also a measure of protection. If, therefore, those whose skins are of this description think that it is necessary to wash in cold water every day in order to keep up to the standard of cleanliness, they remove more than they can spare of this sebaceous material, and leave the skin hard and powdery, and susceptible to all changes of temperature. This may be counteracted in a measure by the use of oil —as salad oil—with which athletes rub themselves after their practising. A very small quantity serves to cover the whole skin, which soon absorbs it. But it is quite a mistake to suppose that frequent washing is necessary to cleanliness. The skin is to a large extent self-clensing, and frequent washing—however pleasant and otherwise desirable it may be—is not a necessity under ordinary conditions. Frequent change of underclothing answers the same purpose as frequent bathing in those whose skins are not very active. For them, a hot bath or a Turkish bath once a week is quite sufficient.

It has been said that the most cleanly people in the world are the poor and the rich. The latter have all the means of washing themselves without the necessity of exertion: the former are obliged to exert themselves in order to earn their living, and their own exertions create that activity of the skin which makes it cleanse itself; whilst the intermediate class, which has not yet attained to the luxury of baths and bath-rooms, and is not compelled to make great muscular exertions, is less cleanly than either. Like most generalizations this contains a good deal of truth, though it won't bear applying in particular instances. There are people who are both poor and lazy, and laziness is the great parent of uncleanliness everywhere.

But apart from the *secretions* of the skin, there is the *circulation* to be considered. There are some whose skins are always chilly in cold weather and ready to develop chilblains, and others who can never get a reaction after a cold bath. These should content themselves with a quick dry-rubbing every morning with a rough towel, and should not think of taking cold baths.

CHAPTER III.

COLD-PREVENTING.

IN discussing the question of cold-catching, the other question of cold-*avoiding* comes in as a matter of course. To all persons about to take cold in the ways above mentioned, the laconic advice of *Mr. Punch* comes naturally to our minds—*don't*. But unhappily we cannot always choose our circumstances, and therefore it is desirable to fortify ourselves against the contingencies alluded to. And, fortunately, there is much to be done in the way of COLD-PREVENTING.

One of the chief precautions against cold is the avoidance of "coddling." The muffler is a great snare. It is much better to accustom the neck to bear a certain amount of exposure, giving it the protection of collar and tie, but nothing more. Sometimes the muffler is relied on as the sole extra wrap on a cold day. If a child has a few yards of knitted stuff twisted around its neck, the fond parent is apt to feel that there is no need to attend to its back and chest. But the muffler will not fill the part of an overcoat, which is the garment really needed.

In speaking of the morning bath,

I have indicated its usefulness for this purpose in those whose constitutions are suitable. And I have also pointed out the value of inunction with oil, such as salad oil, in those whose skins are poor. A very small quantity, about a teaspoonful, will suffice to go over the whole body. If this is done at night, and a woollen sleeping dress worn, the cold bath may be taken without risk and with advantage in the morning, provided there is good reaction. If the reaction is not good, a dry-rubbing must suffice. In children who are chilly and liable to colds, nothing is better than inunction every night with *cod liver oil.* They must, of course, be wrapped in flannel night-dresses.

The odor is not of the pleasantest, but the good effect is so great that this is a small consideration. The child may be sponged in the morning, and briskly rubbed before dressing, and no unpleasant odour will then be detected.

There is another substitute for the morning tub which will probably be found more acceptable to many than the last named, and that is sponging with spirit of wine. Contact with water increases chilliness, but contact with spirit diminishes it. One or two tablespoonfuls of spirit of wine may be poured into a saucer and taken up with a small sponge. This may then be passed rapidly all over the body, and the clothes immediately put on.

The spirit dries at once, so there is no need of towelling afterwards. The effect of this is to impart a feeling of warmth which not unfrequently lasts the entire day. This is especially valuable to those who are excessively sensitive to the effects of damp.

In the prevention of colds, nothing is of greater importance than the question of CLOTHING.

In a changeable climate like that of our country, persons who are at all susceptible to changes in the temperature and weather should be so clothed that they are in a constant state of preparation. There are some who have such active circulations that their skins are never chilly whatever the state of the atmosphere may be. These have a natural defence, and need take no special precautions. They may wear what they like best—cotton, or silk, or wool. But these are the fortunate few. Others who are less highly endowed should wear next their skin, and completely encasing their bodies, a material which will retain the bodily heat and electricity, whilst allowing the escape of the perspiration, much of which comes away in the form of watery vapour. The best of all material of this kind is wool. Dr. Jaeger deserves the thanks of all for the attention he has given to this subject, although like most men with hobbies he is apt to ride his too hard. A complete suit of woollen underclothing is the best possible protection against sudden chilling. And the night-dress may be made of the same material if there is any occasion to be about at night or any difficulty in keeping warm.

There are some whose skins are so sensitive that they cannot endure the contact of wool in any form. For them silk is the best. But silk is not so warm as wool, and not so efficient a protection.

CHAPTER IV.

COLD-CURING.

THERE is a German saying to this effect: "A clever physician will cure a cold in a fortnight; it will get well of itself in fourteen days." The proverb does not venture to say how long a cold will go on under the ministrations of a physician who is *not* clever, or to what length it will run when under amateur treatment. I cannot answer for what may happen in Germany, but I have known colds run on to portentious length under amateur or non-skilful medical guidance in this country. And even physicians of repute sometimes experience no small difficulty in getting rid of a severe catarrh in their own persons. But this proverb was no doubt invented before Hahnemann and his system saw the light. Armed with his therapeutic weapons and a sound judgment, the physician of to-day can bid even colds defiance, and can shorten their fortnight's right of duration by many days.

The value of a therapeutic system and the proficiency of a physician are shown most of all in little things. A system which can only be applied in formidable illness, such as cholera and scarlet fever, is of only limited use in practical life, and a doctor who can only apply it in grave illnesses, and can do nothing in the presence of a cold in the head or an eruption on the face, will find himself a helpless creature in nine-tenths of the cases he is consulted about. Nor is it of much use for him to pooh-pooh all illnesses that do not happen to be attended with danger to life, as some doctors are wont to do,—unless, indeed, they happen to be themselves the patients. Little illnesses deserve just as much attention as the great ones: for though they may not threaten life itself, they do often destroy all its pleasure; and they are much more common than the others. The doctor who affects to despise the minor ills is generally (whether he knows it or not) merely covering his own want of skill and want of knowledge. He does not know what to do with the patient, and so tries to persuade him that the disorder is, as Mr. Toots would say, "of no consequence"—in fact, is quite beneath the range of his great studies, and therefore cannot be worth the notice of any learned mind. But the patient, who is perpetually worried with it, is not so easy to persuade that his toothache, or his headache, or his eruption, or his cold in the head is really nothing, if he can only bring his mind to think so. He only concludes that it is no use taking his complaint to the members of the high and mighty faculty, and betakes himself to old dames' remedies, or quack nostrums whose obliging proprietors promise in their advertisements attention to the most trivial details.

But Homœopathy has brought a vast change into medicine in regard to its general applicability. It can be adapted to any disorder, no matter how grave or how apparently trivial. It is like the steam-hammer, which can crack a nutshell without injuring the nut, or tap a watch-case without breaking it, just as easily as it can weld and shape masses of iron presenting a resisting power of many tons. There are few sensations more pleasant than to awake in the morning and find one's self free from a cold, when the night before one had gone to bed sneezing and shivering, and had abandoned one's self to a fortnight's misery. Thanks to homœopathy and its discoverer, this miracle is performed every day. There is no medicine that will cure every cold, since, as I have pointed out, colds differ widely in their characters. But the homœopathic Materia Medica is so rich that it has a medicine for every one's cold, though it depends on the skill and judgment of the prescriber to find the right one.

Before discussing the homœopathic remedies for cold, and pointing out their leading characteristics and indications, I will speak of the general measures which are resorted to, and often with success.

Nearly every one has his own treatment for his own cold. One will keep himself a prisoner in his house until it is better. Another, as soon as he finds he has taken cold, will take a ten-mile walk at full-speed, and when he comes in go straight to bed, piling on the blankets in order to keep up the effect. A third, before retiring, will mix himself a stiff glass of toddy, and by the time it is finished will at any rate have forgotten his cold, if he has not cured it. The "night-cap treatment," I am reminded by a friend, is sometimes very successful. Night-caps are seldom worn nowadays;

and if one who is not accustomed to them puts one on when he has a cold (or, which comes to the same thing, wraps his head up warmly when he goes to bed), he will often get rid of it by this means. Another efficacious remedy is the time-honoured jorum of hot onion gruel. The more efficient part of the gruel is the onion which it contains, and which we shall see presently (under its botanical name *Cepa* or *Allium cepa*), is strikingly homœopathic to colds. The idea of these remedies (and to them may be added the hot bath and the Turkish bath) is to restore bodily heat, and by perspiration to relieve the internal congestion which has resulted from chilling of the surface and driving the blood inwards. And not unfrequently these measures are quite successful. There is another means of curing colds, and that is what may be called the salt treatment. Later on I shall have occasion to refer to the value of salt as a homœopathic remedy for colds under the name it has always borne in Homœopathy, *Natrum muriaticum.* The ordinary salt treatment for cold consists in eating highly salted food, such as herrings, or visiting salt-mines and salt-baths like those at Droitwich in England, and Ems, Obersalzbrunnen, and Gleichenberg in Germany.

The effects of these salt-springs may be obtained without visiting the locality, by drinking the waters mixed in equal proportions with hot skim-milk or whey. Ems water drunk in this way will often assist the resolution of a cold.

Sulphur-springs, as those of the Eaux-bonnes of the Pyrenees, are valuable for chronic colds of a certain kind. But the same patients who benefit by them would not benefit by the salt-springs; and the constitutional peculiarities of the patient must be considered before the decision is come to about which place to visit.

These extreme measures will, of course, not be thought of for ordinary colds; but only where they have become chronic, and the general health so depraved that ordinary measures are unequal to the task of bringing about the needed constitutional changes.

For constitutions *can* be changed. It is not enough for a doctor to be able to " understand " his patient's constitution—he must be able to alter it sometimes. We often see this effect produced by natural causes. After severe fevers a patient liable to certain forms of illness, such as chest disorder, becomes entirely free from them. It is quite common to hear the remark that " So-and-so has been quite different, and very much better than he used to be, ever since he had the measles," or some other fever. But the change is not always for the better, by any means.

The same fever which will cure a constitutional tendency to disease in one patient, will set up a new one in another.

Following on the lines of Nature, it is possible for us, without setting up a disease, to change the constitutional habit of a patient by a course of treatment; and it is in cases where this is desired, that it is often advantageous to make use of natural mineral springs.

But this is by no means always a necessity. In the appropriate homœopathic remedy we have an agent as powerful for this purpose as the mineral waters where they issue from their fountains.

In the matter of foods, it is found that all greasy kinds act injuriously in catarrhal conditions, and should, therefore, be avoided; whilst salt foods, as salt herrings, are good.

CHAPTER V.

THE MEDICINAL TREATMENT OF ACUTE COLDS.

THE MEDICINAL TREATMENT of colds divides itself naturally into three parts,—Treatment of the *acute attack;* treatment of the *condition* when it has become *chronic;* and treatment of the *constitutional tendency* to be affected by chills.

COLDS IN THE ACUTE STAGE.—Among the remedies for a cold in the incipient stage, two stand out prominently from all the rest—*Camphor* and *Aconite*. There is no remedy that has made more converts to Homœopathy than *Aconite*, and its beautiful effect in dissipating the consequences of a chill is one of the most striking of its virtues. In a certain proportion of patients *Camphor* has an equally marked good effect; but *Camphor* has not such a wide range as its sister drug. Still, *Camphor* must not be neglected. The chill of *Camphor* is more marked than that of *Aconite;* and if a pilule (one of the large pilules sold in stoppered bottles by homœopathic chemists) is taken every fifteen minutes from the moment that the chill has been experienced, and continued for a few hours until the reaction sets in, a cold will almost invariably be warded off. Later on, *Camphor*, though it may prove useful, is not so likely to do so as is *Aconite*. *Aconite** may be taken every hour, in doses of one drop or six pilules, for the first five or six hours, and afterwards

* *N.B.*—In choosing a remedy it is not necessary that the case to be cured should have all the symptoms put down as characteristic of it. It will be sufficient if a few of the leading features of the cold correspond with those of the drug. For instance, a patient suffering from an ordinary cold in the head in the freely running stage took *Mercurius*, and the following day his cold had vanished. It will be found that under *Mercurius* many other symptoms are put down. These are all characteristic of the remedy, and will guide to the choice of it when found in any patient; but it is not necessary to have them all before prescribing the drug.

every two hours. This may be kept up for forty-eight hours.

The use of these two drugs as indicated—*Camphor* when the chill is first taken, *Aconite* if this stage has passed — may be followed, unless there are special reasons why they should not be used, as a routine practice. The great majority of colds will be cut short by them. If *Aconite* causes perspiration, care should be taken to avoid another chill whilst the perspiration is going on. Otherwise, no special precautions need be observed.

It is useless to cite examples of the triumphs of these two medicines, for they are to be found in nearly every family throughout the land;

for the use of *Aconite* in colds is by no means confined to homœopathic practice. The allopaths have in some mysterious way discovered the virtues of the drug, and made free use of it. Many patients of mine regularly cut short their colds with *Aconite* since they have learned how to take it.

If a cold has lasted more than two days, other medicines must be thought of. Among these *Gelsemium*, *Mercurius*, *Arsenicum*, *Nux vomica*, *Pulsatilla*, *Sanguinaria*, *Cepa*, *Natrum muriaticum* hold the first rank, and will be given according as the symptoms they have produced in the healthy correspond to the symptoms of the cold.

Sometimes the fever following

a chill does not yield to *Aconite*, and then *Gelsemium* is generally successful. The symptoms which call for *Gelsemium* are:—Chills creeping up the back, fulness of the head, heat of the face, beating of the arteries in the neck, hot, dry hands, feeling of languor and drowsiness. The restlessness is less intense than that of *Aconite*, and it often subsides without inspiration, and returns again (of the "remitting" type, as it is called). The chilliness is often accompanied by a profuse flow of urine, which relieves the head. With this there is sneezing, fulness at the root of the nose, and flow of clear water from the nose and eyes. Dose: 3^x, one drop or six pilules every hour.

When the nasal discharge is thin and irritating, with a hot burning sensation in nose and eyes, *Arsenicum* is the remedy; and if, in addition, there is burning thirst, red tongue, headache, sleeplessness, anxiety, and prostration, *all the symptoms being ameliorated by warmth*, the indications will be still stronger. The medicine should be given in the 3rd dilution, two drops (or two pilules) every hour or two.

Arsenicum is the best remedy, in a general way, for the "influenza cold," which produces a good deal of prostration, with free, irritating, thin discharge from nose and eyes.

Mercurius is to be given in most common colds when there is an abundant flow of serous mucus from the nose, which is often swollen and red; fetid smell of nasal mucus; heavy frontal headache; deafness; nightly sweats with febrile chill and heat; great thirst; pains in the limbs; low spirits and longing for solitude, *all the symptoms being increased both by heat and cold.* Dose: No. 6, two drops or six pilules every two hours.

Hepar sulph.—When *Mercurius* is indicated, but does not respond, or when the patient has already had too much; when each draught of cold air produces fresh cold or a headache, only one nostril being affected, and the headache being made worse by movement. Dose:

No. 6, two drops or pilules six every two hours.

Cepa (made from the red onion).—Fluent coryza; tightness at root of nose; constant sneezing; pain in back, and chills; melancholy, anxiety, restlessness. Symptoms worse in a room, better out of doors. Dose: No. 3, two drops or six pilules every two hours.

A case of violent cold in the head, with streaming eyes and nose, in a gouty patient, who had also a troublesome irritation of the skin, was cured completely by a few doses of *Cepa*. Usually her attacks, when occurring in the beginning of winter, went on to bronchitis, and in this instance the bronchial tubes had already become affected when I gave the *Cepa*, which cleared off everything.

Pulsatilla.—Discharge of yellowish-green fetid mucus from the nose; loss of appetite and sense of taste; head heavy and embarrassed, especially in the evening and by the warmth of a room, with stoppage of the nose; no thirst; tearful humour; chilliness all the evening; *amelioration in the open air.* Dose: 3^x, two drops or six pilules every two hours.

Nux vomica is the remedy when the cold is "dry" and the nose blocked; or it may be dry in the morning and fluent in the evening. There is heaviness of the forehead. An angry, quarrelsome humour is characteristic of *Nux*. *Aggravation* of symptoms occurs from mental exertion; in the morning;

after retiring, especially after dinner; from motion; from slight touch; in the open air (in this contrasting with *Pulsatilla*, as it does in so many points); and in dry weather.

Sanguinaria or *Nitrate of Sanguinarin.*—Profuse fluent coryza; or dry, with frequent sneezing; dull, heavy pain at the root of the nose; odour of roasted onions in the nose; dryness of lips; tongue feels as if burnt; throat full, swollen, and constricted; sharp stitches in chest; depression and irritability. *Aggravation: morning and evening; from light and motion.* Dose of *Sanguinaria:* No. 1, two drops or six pilules every two hours. Of *Nitrate of Sanguinarin*, 3^x

trituration, one grain every two hours.

Natrum muriaticum. — Fluent coryza in chilly subjects; chills along the back; great thirst; vesicles on the lips or tendency to them; constipation; weight in forehead on rising in the morning; sadness, depression, tendency to weep. *Aggravation of symptoms in the morning, and periodically.* Dose: 3 trit., two grains every two hours; or No. 6, two drops or six pilules every two hours.

I take some credit to myself for bringing forward *Natrum muriaticum* as a remedy for colds. About sixteen years ago, when Dr. Burnett's work on the drug appeared, I made a study of it, and was struck with the number of cold-symptoms it possessed. Having a pretty severe cold myself at the time, I took a few doses of No. 6, and was intensely delighted to find my cold quite cured in the morning. I soon repeated the happy experience on several patients; and then my partner, Dr. W. Roche, gave it on my recommendation to a patient of his own who was suffering from a very severe cold. This patient declared he had never got rid of a cold so quickly in his life. At that time I thought that the range of the drug was so wide that it was equal to curing almost any cold. Subsequent experience did not justify that, but it did confirm me in my opinion that it is one of the most valuable remedies for cold we possess. It was whilst reading up the literature of this drug that I was struck by the coincidence of its being also recommended, from the old school point of view, in the shape of salt baths or douches; and also by the popular use of the drug in salt food I shall have to refer to it again as a remedy for chronic colds and the cold-constitution.

Kali hydriodicum (*Iodide of Potassium*).—Profuse flow of clear water from eyes and nose; accumulation of thick, tenacious mucus in the nose; discharge of greenish-black or yellow matter of foul smell; nose-bleed; discharge of decomposed greenish-red blood. Sensation of fulness and tightness at the root of the nose; swelling and redness of the nose; sensation of fulness in the nose; with beating pains in the nasal bones; throbbing and burning in nasal and frontal bone with swelling; after abuse of mercury. *Aggravation: at night; in cold air; at rest; better from motion.* Dose: No. 3 or 30, two drops or six pilules every two hours.

These are the chief medicines that will be required for the cure of ACUTE COLDS.

CHAPTER VI.

THE MEDICINAL TREATMENT OF CATARRH OR CHRONIC COLDS AND THE TENDENCY TO TAKE COLD.

CHRONIC COLDS require somewhat different treatment. When a cold has gone on for weeks without any signs of passing away, Turkish baths, hot baths, hot foot baths, warm gruel, and all the rest of the domestic armamentarium having proved in vain, there is still some hope for the unhappy sufferer. He may yet find deliverance from the ruthless enemy which holds him by the nose, without going to a warm climate or waiting till the summer comes.

If the patient has not been already under homœopathic treatment, the remedy for the case will most likely be found among those already described after *Camphor* and *Aconite;* and even if he has had homœopathic treatment, and his symptoms correspond to those which are characteristic of any one of the above-named remedies, this must be given.

The chief remedies for chronic colds are *Hydrastis*, *Calc. carb.*, *Natrum mur.*, *Dulcamara*, *Mercurius*, *Sulphur*.

Hydrastis.—This remedy is indicated when there is much thick discharge from the nose, and especially the posterior part of the nose which leads to the throat; when the mucus drops down into the throat, which is also affected with the catarrhal condition; tongue yellow-coated; tendency to constipation. Dose: No. 1, two drops or six pilules every two hours.

Hydrastis will be found useful in many conditions. A patient who suffered from chronic cold in the nose, and also deafness (which latter was the result of scarlatina, and dated many years back), the discharge from the nose being thick and the throat being also affected, was completely cured of the catarrh by a course of *Hydrastis*, the deafness being also slightly improved. When a cold has settled in the back of the nose and throat, with a good deal of phlegm in the throat, and perhaps deafness, there is no better remedy than *Hydrastis.*

Calcarea carb.—In persons of phlegmatic temperament, pale, and inclined to be fat; in fair, plump children; in persons who suffer from acidity; internal chilliness; coryza, chiefly dry; nostrils sore; polypus; margins of eyelids sore. *Aggravation: mornings, evenings, and after midnight; from cold and cold air.* Dose: No. 6, two drops or six pilules every four hours.

Natrum mur.—When the coryza is fluent; chilly subjects; the blood thin and watery; complexion unhealthy; thirst; constipation.

Disposition melancholy and tearful. Dose: No. 6, two drops or six pilules every two hours. It is patients of this description who will benefit by brine baths The baths should be hot, and should not be stayed in too long. They should be followed by cold spraying.

Dulcamara.—Extreme sensitiveness to damp cold; blocking of the nose, with a discharge that the least cold air stops anew; dryness of the mouth without thirst; hoarseness. *Aggravation: during rest; amelioration during movement.* Dose: No. 6, two drops or six pilules every two hours.

Mercurius.—Abundant thick or fluent coryza of fetid odor; feverish condition; night sweats; pains in the limbs; desire for solitude. *Aggravation by both heat and cold.* Dose: No. 3^x trit., two grains, or two drops of No. 6, every four hours.

Sulphur.—Blocking and great dryness of the nose, or abundant secretion of thick, yellowish, purulent mucus; bleeding; loss of smell; suited to lean persons inclined to stoop; those subject to skin affections who perspire easily. *Aggravation from warmth of bed and during rest; better during motion and when walking.* Dose: No. 6, two drops or six pilules every two hours.

It is sometimes advisable to send patients of the sulphur type, if the English climate tries them greatly, to the sulphur springs, such as those of Eaux-Bonnes in the Pyrenees.

Among the sequelæ of a cold in the head (vulgarly called "dregs of a cold") may be mentioned loss of taste and smell. This sometimes persists for a long time after all other signs of a cold have disappeared. For this the remedy is *Magnes. mur.* 6, two drops or six pilules every four hours.

The TENDENCY TO TAKE COLD may be counteracted by a course of constitutional treatment. In order that this may be brought about, every individual must be considered in the light of his own constitutional peculiarities. Only the remedies most generally applicable can be indicated here, but they will be found to cover a very large number of cases.

The remedies should be taken

steadily twice or three times a day, and should be continued for one or two months. They may be commenced, if indicated, whilst the cold still continues, or after it is cured.

The remedies I shall name in this connexion are *Natrum mur.*, *Calc. carb.*, *Carbo veg.*, *Agaricus*, *Sulphur*, *Mercurius.* These remedies must be selected according as they correspond with the constitutional state of the patient, rather than with any idea of finding an agreement between their cold symptoms and the peculiar features of the patients' colds when they have them.

Natrum mur.—Anæmic, ill-nourished, chilly persons, of unclear complexions; inclined to constipation; despondent and tearful; feel worse when lying down, from heat; better in open air. Dose: No. 12, two drops or six pilules three times a day.

With this remedy I have frequently removed the susceptibility to cold. Here is a case typical of many. A young girl about puberty, subject to colds, which came on with a kind of bilious attack; always chilly; hands and feet never warm, clammy; of nervous temperament; and somewhat anæmic. *Nat. mur.* 12, six pilules night and morning, made a complete revolution in her general health and susceptibility to chills within a month.

Calc. carb.—Pale, phlegmatic persons; abnormally fat young people; scrofulous or tubercular tendency;

those liable to acidity. Feel worse from cold and cold air. Dose: No. 12, two drops or six pilules three times a day.

Carbo veg.—Persons whose vital powers are low; venous system predominant, giving a blue look to the countenance and flesh; cold blue hands and feet; symptoms worse in cold damp weather. Dose: No. 12, two drops or six pilules three times a day.

Agaricus.—When there is marked tendency to chilblains; more suited for persons of light hair and lax fibre, and for old persons with indolent circulation. Symptoms worse in night; in cold air; during repose; before a thunderstorm. Dose: No. 6, two drops or six pilules three times a day.

Sulphur.—Chilly persons with tendency to skin irritation or actual skin disease; tendency to constipation and piles; symptoms being worse from warmth and by rest. Dose: No. 30, one drop or six pilules three times a day.

Mercurius.—Scrofulous, rheumatic, bilious persons, and those subject to catarrhs of all kinds; broken down constitutions; trembling limbs; cold pale hands and feet. *Patients feel worse at night from warmth of bed; from perspiration; cold weather; cold evening air; warm autumn days; damp cold nights; better during the day and during rest.* Dose: No. 12, two drops or six pilules three times a day.

CHAPTER VII.

NASAL POLYPUS.

ONE of the consequences of chronic irritation of the nasal mucous membrane is the development of polypus, which consists of an immensely hypertrophied follicle of normal mucous membrane. There are also polypi, which consist of new growth, arising independently of chronic irritation or catarrh, but I am only dealing here with the simple and commoner kind.

A polypus may exist some time without giving rise to any symptoms; but when it increases so far as to obstruct the passage of air through the nose and into the lungs, a great deal of discomfort and annoyance is occasioned. The patient is often aroused in the middle of the night with distressing sensations of suffocation. Attacks of spasmodic asthma may occur. The nose being the upper extremity of the air passages, the lungs are in intimate nervous sympathy with it, and affections of the nose often produce symptoms in the lungs.

Polypi sometimes have their origin in the anterior part of the nasal mucous membrane, and when of any size they can be seen as red moist masses on looking into the nostrils. Sometimes they are further back, and hang into the back of the throat. They are almost always attended with copious discharge, both front and back, keeping up a continual "cold."

The usual method of dealing with polypus is to remove it, and the method now most approved is by the electric wire. But polypus is a constitutional affair, and should by right be cured by constitutional remedies. This has been done times out of number, and should always be aimed at by homœopathists.

A year or two ago I was consulted by letter on behalf of a young lady, aged 20, in the country, who had been troubled for three or four years with an excessive discharge from the nose and dropping of discharge from back of the nose down the throat. The least cold air aggravated the complaint, and, conversely, it was better in a warm room. She suffered, in addition, from cold, damp feet; faint feelings, and bilious sick headaches.

She received *Calcarea* in very high potencies at rare intervals. From the first the symptoms began to improve. Later on, *Thuja* was given, and afterwards *Dulcamara*, *Silica*, and *Stannum*, her health and the local symptoms steadily improving all the time. About eighteen months from the commencement of the course she passed from the nose a polypus an inch and a half in length. The passing was preceded and followed by sharp bleeding. There has been no recurrence since.

It may be objected that the treatment occupied a long time, whereas an operation could have relieved the patient in a few minutes. This is true so far as the removal of the polypus is concerned, but the effect of the medicinal treatment was to bring about a complete constitutional change in the patient, and to work a constitutional cure. Polypi have an awkward habit of recurring after removal by operation; but when a cure is wrought by medicine the tendency to recur is removed. Moreover, operative removal of a polypus does not cure the original irritation which gave rise to the formation as constitutional treatment does.

The remedies chiefly credited with the cure of polypus are *Calcarea* (which had a leading share in my case), and *Thuja* (which was also used), *Nitric acid*, *Sanguinaria*, *Phosphorus*, and *Teucrium*. Lately, Dr. Cooper has introduced a new remedy, *Lemna minor*, the well-known duckweed, which has effected remarkable cures in his own practice and that of others, and which promises to be a very important medicine in nasal cases. Cases of atrophic rhinitis have been reported as cured by it. Aggravation in damp weather is a leading indication for its use.

The indications for the different remedies mentioned above will be found in the *Materia Medica* at the end of the work.

CHAPTER VIII.

HAY FEVER.

IN the early summer, just when the grass is in flower, a number of people become affected with violent irritation of the nasal mucous membrane, accompanied with more or less constitutional disturbance, as prostration and fever, with catarrh, congestion of the eyes, headache, oppression of the breathing. This condition lasts throughout the summer whenever the individual comes in contact with the effluvia of hay. The symptoms are caused by particles of the pollen of the hay which find their way into the nasal cavities. Hay is not the only offender, as the pollen of many flowers is capable of setting up the same train of symptoms,—violent and almost incessant sneezing, streaming eyes and nostrils, chilliness and feverish symptoms, headache, and often great depression, general weakness, and wasting.

How is it, it may be asked, seeing that the pollen is everywhere inhaled by everybody, that all are not affected alike? The reply, that not all persons are sensitive alike, brings us to the further query, Why are some sensitive and others not? Here we arrive at the crux of the whole matter: it is a constitutional weakness of some kind or other, and in numberless cases I have traced it to that great parent of woes—GOUT. I have known many persons, members of highly gouty families, who have prided themselves on being the only ones who have escaped gout, when all the time they have had it in their noses without recognizing it. For my part, I consider it less objectionable in the toe.

Gout, in my experience, constitutes a large section of the great psoric family of disorders as classified by Hahnemann. But in many subjects of hay fever, it is sycosis, the second of the disease-miasms described by Hahnemann, which is at the root of the disorder.

Though only manifest in the summer, the disease actually exists through the winter, only awaiting the peculiar stimulus to make it manifest. Careful observation of a patient in the intervals of the attacks will disclose the nature of the constitutional tendency.

It is astonishing to what shifts those who have the means to adopt them are driven to escape their summer enemy. In flight to the high Alps some find safety; but the safest place of all is on board ship. But homœopathic treatment can, in a large number of cases, save the necessity of yearly banishment; and even when it cannot altogether prevent the recurrence of attacks, it can so far mitigate their severity as to render life just tolerable in spite of them.

A few years ago, in the early summer, I was consulted by a gentleman, aged 40, who had been subject to hay fever from May till August every year as long as he could remember. He had had very severe treatment for it, including operations on the bones of his nose and cauterising the mucous membrane with electric cauteries. Still the attacks were no better. In a very short time antipsoric treatment put an end to all the symptoms. He passed through the summer without any trouble, and he has hardly had any to speak of since.

Naphthalin 3^x (one drop or six pilules every two hours) has proved itself a very useful remedy in a large number of cases.

Sabadilla 3 (every two or four hours), violent sneezing with lachrymation, redness and swelling of eyelids, contractions, stupefying headache.

Arsenicum 3, with thirst, fever, restlessness and anguish; aggravation from cold air. This may be given every two hours during an attack, and twice a day beforehand as a prophylactic.

Psorinum 30 will cure a large number of cases when there is very great sensitiveness to cold. Patients like to be near a fire or wrapped in furs even in summer weather. It may be given three or four times a day.

SECTION II.

Gripipe or Influenza.

CHAPTER I.

DESCRIPTION.

SINCE the earlier editions of this book were written the worst epidemic of Influenza within modern times has visited all parts of the civilised world, and seems to demand some notice in a treatise on colds, especially as we are not yet by any means rid of the disease, and may at any time find ourselves face to face with a fresh outbreak.

In order to distinguish it from the "Influenza Colds," which we have always with us, the malady is sometimes called "Siberian" or "Russian" Influenza, since the epidemics have always begun in the northern part of the Russian Empire. Corresponding to its chilly origin, one of the features of the disease is to cause an intense chilliness, alternating with fever, and to leave the patient excessively sensitive to cold for a very long time after. Many persons who have never before required or even tolerated woollen clothing next the skin have been compelled to adopt it after undergoing an attack. In this respect it is like the malarial fevers, and some have on this account given it the name "malarial catarrh." But it is clearly distinguished from true malaria by its infectious character. The poison of ague is obviously of earth and water origin, and when a person has contracted ague in a malarial district, and afterwards leaves that district and has an attack of ague, he does not communicate the disease to others. Influenza, whatever may be its origin, certainly does spread from one person to another by direct infection. But here again is a peculiarity : it has no fixed period of development, and there is no certainty of its developing at all. Some persons have been struck down within an hour or two after exposure to infection. Others have gone days, and have only been affected when they have "caught cold," the chill having the effect of lowering the vitality, and giving the poison the opportunity of developing. This explains how it is that elaborate precautions for avoiding infection have not been of much use. In the height of an epidemic the infection is probably everywhere. Every person has the germs in him, but it requires some exciting cause to rouse them into activity. When a person becomes infected with small-pox, for instance, within a fortnight the disease will appear. It requires no additional impetus to start it into life; and so it is with all the eruptive fevers. But with influenza it is very different. The poison may be dormant for an indefinite time, and may show itself after the person has been exposed to a chill, a wetting, an overstrain of any kind, or an accident.

The *forms* which influenza may take are protean. There is no one symptom that I know of that is common to all, or even to the majority of cases. Some people think it necessary for there to be rise of temperature; that unless there is fever it cannot be influenza. I have seen many cases of unmistakable influenza in which the temperature has been all the time subnormal.

The classical type of influenza is marked by severe pains and soreness all over, especially in the back and head, and frequently setting in quite suddenly. Repeated chills are followed by high fever, with increase of the pains. The eyes are bleery, the intellect dulled, and a sleepy, heavy condition induced. There is a heavy nasal catarrh, which persists long after the acute symptoms have passed off. The tongue is foul; appetite lost. The throat is generally inflamed, and with all there is great prostration and mental depression. The pulse is as often slow as frequent, and does not correspond to the temperature. The attack may last from one to several days.

This is the classical type, but the departures from it are innumerable. It may attack the chest, the heart, the bowels, or the brain. To describe them all would require a treatise on almost all the diseases that exist, for there is hardly any disease that influenza will not take the form of.

In fact, one of the great predisposing factors to an attack of influenza is a constitutional weakness of some kind. Gout is one of its favourite bases. Influenza very readily combines with gout, and aggravates every gouty manifestation a patient may have had before, whether it be a skin affection, joint-pains, catarrh, or any other of the innumerable expressions of the gouty diathesis.

One attack of the disease has no

effect in protecting against a second, and, on the contrary, it seems rather to predispose to it. Relapses are very frequent. In many cases it seems as if recovery was never quite complete, the poison being always in the system, and ready to be excited to activity by any lowering cause. These cases require the most persistent and patient constitutional treatment to restore them to health. And the same may be said of the consequences which influenza leaves behind in the shape of neuralgias, sciatica, nervous breakdown (or "neurasthenia" as it is now the fashion to call it), mental depression, and heart weakness and irritability, of which every practitioner has seen so much since the epidemic appeared. In these cases it is often impossible to succeed, unless the patient can be persuaded to submit to a period of absolute rest. The general rule is, that as soon as they gather an amount of strength—feeling better—patients want to spend it. If they do, they soon drop down into the lowest depths again.

CHAPTER II.

TREATMENT.

THE treatment of influenza is as various as its forms. The best preventive is to keep well-fed, well-clothed; to avoid chilling, wetting, and exhaustion in any form, especially over-fatigue, or going too long without food. Many remedies have been recommended as prophylactics, especially *Ammoniated Quinine* and *Eucalyptus*, the odour of which last was at one time universally prevalent in every public place. I do not advise the use of either. In my experience the best preventive is *Arsenicum.* Six pilules of *Arsenicum* in the No. 3 strength should be taken three times a day when the epidemic is about.

What about going to bed? In severe cases this question needs no answer—the patient simply cannot stay up. But in a number of others the patient has strength enough to keep going on—is he to do it? Wherever there is a doubt it should be decided in favour of bed. It is true many persons have fought through an attack without seeming to take harm from it; but wherever there is any delicacy of constitution, or where an internal organ has become inflamed, delay in going to bed is attended with great danger. Every case must be decided on its own merits.

The routine practice should be: Rest in bed, with hot bottles to feet if they are cold; light nourishment, as gruel, beef-tea, mutton broth or chicken tea, or milk diluted with boiling water, every two or three hours. This should be kept up till the fever goes, and the tongue becomes clean, and the appetite returns. As soon as the patient can eat, he should have all the nourishment he can be got to take.

With regard to baths, the caution given in an earlier chapter must be emphasized here. Complete baths are to be avoided, and blanket baths only are to be allowed. That is to say, the patient is to be rolled in a blanket, and sponged with hot water in detachments, each part being dried with a hot towel before another is washed. A complete bath should not be indulged in till recovery is complete; many a relapse has been occasioned by neglect of this rule.

Medicines.

I have already mentioned that *Arsenicum* is the best prophylactic medicine I know. The nearest to a specific for the disease is *Baptisia.* It has all the symptoms described above in the classical type; the general aching and soreness, heavy head, besotted appearance, loaded tongue, sore throat, and fever,—and if no other remedy is clearly indicated in preference, I should give *Bapt.* every hour. It is effective in all attenuations. I prefer the 30th; but others have used the tincture with success, and all dilutions between. For general practice one or two drop doses of the 3^x is perhaps the best.

Among other medicines may be named the following, with their leading indications:—

Aconite.—Sharp fever; dry skin; great restlessness; depression; anguish; sense of impending death. No. 3, one or two drops or six pilules every hour.

Belladonna.—Intense throbbing headache, highly flushed face, tendency to delirium; thirst, sore throat. Facial neuralgia and earache, especially right side. No. 3, every hour.

Bryonia.—Where the least movement of any kind aggravates the symptoms. No. 3, every hour.

Rhus tox.—The opposite of *Bry.* The patient cannot keep still; has to move about to relieve the otherwise intolerable pains. Where the attack has been provoked by getting wet. No. 3, every hour.

Gelsemium.—Where paralytic symptoms predominate, especially of the lower limbs. Intense headache; strong full pulse; giddiness. No. 3, every hour.

Phytolacca.—Specific when the throat is inflamed and spotty, the glands externally being hard and tender. No. 3, internally, every hour, and a gargle of the θ tincture —ten drops to a teacupful of water. The gargle may be used every four hours.

China.—When the headache is accompanied by giddiness and noises in the ears. In one case of this kind I relieved a patient—who was driven to the verge of madness by this symptom—in a few minutes with *China* 30, and no other medicine was required.

In the CHRONIC EFFECTS OF INFLUENZA AND RESULTING DEBILITY careful constitutional treatment is required, and each case must be treated by itself. There are, however, a few remedies which may be usefully mentioned here.

Natrum salicylicum, No. 3, every two or four hours, has relieved many cases in which symptoms of vertigo, with noise in the head, have remained after influenza. Patients to whom I have given it have so frequently praised its "tonic" effect that I have given it (and with great success) where the debility has been the leading symptom, and no head symptoms have been complained of. *Sulphur*, *Arsenicum*, and *Natrum mur.* will be frequently required, according to indications already given. In the profound prostration, with loss of flesh, which often follows, *Kali iodatum* 30, every four hours, has proved a very efficient remedy in my experience. Finally, where there is great chilliness, debility that compels the patient to lie down, sinking sensation and general prostration, *Psorinum* 30, three or four times a day, will give great relief.

MATERIA MEDICA.

ACONITE.—Suitable for a cold from the commencement and during the first two days. Influenza.

Symptoms.—Chills and heats, sneezing, coryza, headache. In influenza: sharp fever, dry skin, great depression, and intense restlessness and anxiety.

Dose: No. 3, one drop or six pilules every hour.

AGARICUS.—To correct tendency to colds.

Symptoms.—Chilblains; nervous twitchings; indolent circulation; in persons of light hair and lax fibre; inclined to be fat; feel worse in the night; in cold air; during repose; before a thunderstorm.

Dose: No. 6, two drops or six pilules three times a day.

ARSENICUM.—For acute or chronic colds. Also in hay fever and influenza, both as a prophylactic and in the treatment of the disease when indicated by the symptoms.

Symptoms.—Thin, irritating nasal discharge; hot, burning sensation in nose and eyes; burning thirst; red tongue; anxiety; restlessness; prostration; fever; headache; sleeplessness. Better by warmth.

Dose: No. 3, two drops or six pilules every two hours. As a prophylactic, twice a day.

BAPTISIA.—Almost specific in influenza.

Symptoms.—Pains all over and general soreness; restlessness; drowsy; besotted expression; catarrh; sore throat, headache.

Dose: No. 3^x, one or two drops every hour.

BELLADONNA.—Influenza.

Symptoms.—Intense throbbing headache; highly flushed face; sore throat; tendency to delirium, neuralgia of face, and earache.

Dose: No. 3, one or two drops every hour.

BRYONIA.—Influenza.

Symptoms.—Pains all over, *aggravated by the least movement.*

Dose: No. 3^x, one or two drops every hour.

CALCAREA CARB.—Suitable for chronic colds and for correcting the tendency to colds. Also for Polypus.

Symptoms.—The leuco-phlegmatic temperament; acidity; internal chilliness; coryza, chiefly dry; nostrils sore; polypus; margins of eyelids sore. Aggravation of symptoms morning and evening, from cold water and cold air.

Dose: For chronic cold, No. 6, two drops or six pilules every two hours.

For correcting tendency, No. 12, two drops or six pilules three times a day.

CAMPHOR.—At the very beginning of a cold before the chill has passed off. *Camphor* was recommended by Hahnemann as a remedy for Russian influenza, and has been used with good effect in the recent epidemic, when the initial chill has been great and attended with great prostration.

Dose: One camphor pill, or one drop of Rubini's tincture on sugar, every fifteen minutes until reaction sets in.

CARBO VEG.—For correcting tendency to colds.

Symptoms.—Low vital power; venous engorgement, giving the skin and complexion a blue appearance; blue cold hands and feet; aggravation in warm damp weather.

Dose: No. 12, two drops or six pilules three times a day.

CEPA (*Allium cepa*).—Acute colds.

Symptoms.—Fluent coryza; tightness at root of nose; constant sneezing; pain in back, and chills; melancholy, anxiety, restlessness. Worse entering warm room from cold air; better out of doors.

Dose: No. 3, two drops or six pilules every two hours.

DULCAMARA.—In chronic colds.

Symptoms.—Extreme sensitiveness to damp cold; blocking of the nose, with a discharge which the least cold air stops again; dryness of the mouth without thirst; hoarseness; aggravation during rest; amelioration during movement.

Dose: No. 6, two drops or six pilules every two hours.

GELSEMIUM.—In acute colds. Influenza.

Symptoms.—Creeping chills up the back; fulness of the head; heat of face; fulness over root of nose; sneezing; fluent coryza; restlessness at night, with drowsiness and languor. The fever remits, passing off without perspiration, and recurring again. With the chills there is profuse flow of urine with relief to the head. Aggravation of symptoms by warmth of bed; after midnight; in damp weather; and from change of weather.

Dose : No. 1, one drop or six pilules every hour.

HEPAR.—Acute and chronic colds when *Mercurius* is indicated but fails to act, or where the patient has been overdosed with mercury formerly.

Symptoms.—When each draught of air produces a fresh cold or a headache, the cold affecting one nostril only, and the headache being made worse by movement.

Dose : No. 6, two drops or six pilules every two hours.

HYDRASTIS.—For chronic colds.

Symptoms. — Much thick discharge from the nose, and especially from the posterior part which leads to the throat; mucus dropping down into the throat; throat in catarrhal condition; tongue yellow-coated; constipation; all-gone "sinking" sensation at epigastrium.

Dose: No. 1, two drops or six pilules every two hours.

KALI HYDRIODICUM (*Iodide of Potassium*).—Acute and chronic colds. Influenza and its resulting debility.

Symptoms.—Profuse flow of clear water from eyes and nose; accumulation of thick tenacious mucus in the nose; discharge of greenish-black or yellow matter of foul smell; nose-bleed; discharge of decomposed greenish-red blood; sensation of fulness and tightness at the root of the nose; swelling and redness of the nose; sensation of swelling in the nose, with beating pains in the nasal bones; throbbing and burning in nasal and frontal bones, with swelling; abuse of mercury. Aggravation: at night; in cold air; at rest. Better from motion.

Dose: Nos. 3 or 30, two drops or six pilules every two hours.

LEMNA.—Colds and polypus.

Symptoms.—The indications for this medicine are obstruction of the nose, especially bad in damp weather.

Dose: No. 3^x, two drops three times a day.

MAGNESIA MUR.—For loss of taste and smell left behind after a cold.

Dose: No. 6, two drops every four hours.

MERCURIUS (*Mercurius solubilis* or *Mercurius vivus*).—For acute and chronic colds. Tendency to take cold.

Symptoms.—Common cold, with abundant discharge of serous mucus; nose swollen and red; fetid smell of nasal mucus; heavy frontal headache; deafness; nightly sweat, with febrile chill and heat; great thirst; pain in the limbs; low spirits; desire for solitude; all symptoms increased both by heat and cold.

Dose: For cold, No. 6, two drops or six pilules every two hours. For the liability to cold, No. 12, two drops or six pilules three times a day.

NAPHTHALIN.—Hay fever.

Dose: One drop or six pilules every two hours whilst the acute symptoms last.

NATRUM MUR.—Acute and chronic colds. Liability to cold. Influenza.

Symptoms.—Fluent coryza; weight in forehead on rising in the morning; vesicles on lips; chills along the back; constipation; sadness, depression, inclination to weep; aggravation of symptoms in the morning and periodically; chilly subjects; unclear complexion; after malarial fevers or abuse of quinine; anæmia.

Dose: For colds, No. 6, two drops or six pilules every two hours. For liability to cold, No. 12, two drops or six pilules three times a day.

NATRUM SALICYLICUM.—Debility after influenza.

Symptoms.—Great weakness, with tightness of the head, especially if there is deafness, with giddiness and noises in the ears.

Dose: No. 3, one or two drops four times a day.

NUX VOMICA.—Acute colds.

Symptoms.—Dry coryza, with blocking of the nose; or dry coryza in the morning and fluent in the evening and night; heaviness of forehead; angry and quarrelsome humour; constipation. Aggravation from mental exertion; in the morning; after eating, especially after dinner; from motion; from slight touch; in open air; in dry weather.

Dose: No. 3, two drops or six pilules every two hours.

PHYTOLACCA.—Influenza.

Symptoms.—Sore throat with white spots on tonsils and sore glands externally; pains in the back and all over; worst in damp weather.

Dose: No. 3^x, one or two drops every hour. A gargle of five drops of the θ tincture to a teacupful of water may be used every three or four hours.

PSORINUM.—Chronic colds. Influenza. Hay fever.

Symptoms.—Constant sneezing; dropping of mucus down posterior nares; great aversion to cold air and to washing; prostration; sinking sensation; better lying down. Follows *Sulphur* well.

Dose: No. 30, six pilules three or four times a day.

PULSATILLA.—Acute colds.

Symptoms.—Discharge of yellowish-green fetid mucus; loss of appetite and sense of taste; head heavy and embarrassed, especially in the evening and by warmth of a room, with stopping of the nose; absence of thirst; chilliness in the evening; better in the open air. Suitable for blonde persons; of soft fibre; gentle disposition.

Dose: No. 3, two drops or six pilules every two hours.

RHUS TOX.—Influenza.

Symptoms.—The opposite of *Bryonia.* The patient must move about continually to get relief from pains.

Dose: No. 3, one or two drops every hour.

SABADILLA.—Hay fever.

Symptoms. — Violent sneezing with lachrymation; redness and swelling of eyelids; contracting, stupefying headache.

Dose: No. 3, two drops or six pilules every two hours.

SANGUINARIA CANAD. and NITRATE OF SANGUINARIN.—For acute and chronic colds. Polypus.

Symptoms.—Coryza profuse and fluent; or dry, with frequent sneezing; dull, heavy pain at root of nose; odour of roasted onions in the nose; dryness of lips; tongue feels as if burnt; throat full, swollen, and constricted; sharp stitches in chest; depression and irritability. Aggravation morning and evening; from light and motion.

Dose: Sanguinaria, No. 1, two drops or six pilules every two hours; *Nitrate of Sanguinarin*, No. 3^x trituration, one grain every two hours.

SULPHUR.—For chronic colds and for tendency to colds. Effects of influenza.

Symptoms.—Blocking and great dryness of nose; or abundant secretion of thick, yellowish, purulent mucus; bleeding; loss of smell; tendency to skin affections and to perspire easily. Aggravation from warmth of bed and during rest; better during motion.

Dose: For cold, No. 6, two drops or

six pilules every two hours. For tendency, No. 30, two drops or six pilules three times a day.

THUJA.—Chronic colds. Polypus.

Symptoms.—Sensitiveness to cold and damp; sycotic subjects; in those who have suffered much from vaccination.

Dose: No. 30, a drop or six pilules once a day.

INDEX.